Other Books by Tony Seton

Long Short Fiction Truth
The Larger Reality / The Realm of Higher
Consciousness
Do You Mind? The Ultimate App
Thought So
True Tens / Seven Women of Beautiful Character
The Flight of KAL 007
The Bright Wise Solution
Mokki's Peak
Silent Alarm
Deki-san
Equinox
No Soap, Radio
Paradise Pond
Selected Writings
Jennifer
The Francie LeVillard Mysteries - Volumes I - XI
The Francie LeVillard Mysteries - The Early Years
Trinidad Head
Just Imagine
The Autobiography of John Dough, Gigolo
Silver Lining
Mayhem
The Omega Crystal/New Moves
Truth Be Told
Musings on Sherlock Holmes
Say It Write
Is There a Why?
13 Days of Fear
The Brink
Dead as a Doorbell
The Quality Interview / Getting It Right
       on Both Sides of the Mic
Don't Mess with the Press / How to Write, Produce,
       and Report Quality Television News
Right Car, Right Price

Covid Blue

Covid Blue

by Tony Seton

Carmel, California

September 2025

While the characters and most of the text in this book are fictional, some are only slightly stretched from real events. Mainly the information has been drawn from extensive research about the coronavirus pandemic from many sources including doctors and nurses and other journalists. The two primary characters in these pages are nurse Lucy Balfour and journalist David Skye. They were first introduced in *Silver Lining*, an earlier novel by the author.

Covid Blue

ISBN-13: 978-1-7325450-8-3

Printed in the United States of America

Table of Contents

Covid Blue

The Cast

(In order of appearance)

Lucy Balfour, Nurse; David's life partner

David Skye, Journalist; Lucy's life partner

Lascar, Ambulance driver

Lopez, Ambulance medic

Rose Metafleur, E-R manager

Daughter, of a patient in E-R

Phyllis Clavell, Nurse, Hospital intake manager

Ann, Nurse

Betty, Nurse

Carol, Nurse

Doug, Nurse

Jerome Satay, Board member

Myrna Charles, Dispensary staffer

Meghan Royal, Assistant facilities manager

Wendell Mencken, Psychotherapist

Marty Bevsage, Editorial page editor

Covid Blue

Introductions

LUCY

I'm Lucy Balfour. I've been a nurse for more than fifteen years. My specialty has been seeing directly to patient care. It enabled me to develop a relationship with each person to help them deal with what they were facing and to produce the best results.

Until last year, when the pandemic struck. Before then, before we had even heard of the coronavirus, I loved my work. I was able to provide solace and support for the patients. But in 2020 all the beds were filled all the time. They mostly only became empty when the patient had died from Covid.

It was exceedingly painful for me. In the past, I was always ready to work more hours, to take on more patients. But those patients were going to leave in better health. The patients of the pandemic were going to die. I simply couldn't extend myself. It was hard enough with the regular schedule.

What made the difference was David. Knowing that I would see him, be in his arms, feeling his love, made it possible for me to do what I did. Without knowing that he was at our home, waiting for me, I wouldn't have stayed at the hospital. It was our love that enabled me to stay.

But then with the Delta variant, the stress and strain got impossibly worse. It seemed that there would be no end to it. There would be new variants, maybe even worse than Delta. I would not throw away my life on this pointless struggle. That's when I made the decision to quit.

*   *   *   *   *

DAVID

I'm David Skye. I'm a journalist. A freelancer; not working for anyone at the moment. I don't have to. So my work – and it's a pleasure – is making life easier for my darling, Lucy. She works hard enough for both of us as the widely-acclaimed, finest, patients' nurse in the Santa Marino Hospital.

That's where we met ten years ago. I was a patient having been slightly injured by a stray bullet from a crazy PR stunt that struck a car side mirror and drove a piece of glass into my thigh. Lucy, who looked a lot like Nurse Dish (Jo Ann Pflug) in the film *M*A*S*H,* was at my bedside when I awakened. We had an instant connection. (Great story. You can read about it in the book *Silver Lining.)*

Since the pandemic struck, Lucy's job has been going from worse to agonizing and lately has bordered on impossible. She is as noble and dedicated a person as I have ever known, and I have been doing my best to make her time away from the hospital as recuperative as possible. But I think she has come to the end of her rope.

Covid Blue

Time to Go

Lucy Balfour walks into the house looking like she's had a very long day. Not unusual since she has been working twelve-hour shifts for the past ten days. Her willingness to put in the extra hours is just one of the reasons why she is considered one of the most dedicated nurses in the Santa Marino Hospital.

David Skye meets her at the door, taking her into his arms and pushing the door closed behind her. She lets him hold her for what seemed like forever, and then she tilts her head back and looks into his eyes with a widening smile.

LUCY

It is heaven, to be in your arms, my darling. And I know. I came from hell.

David puts his arm around her and leads her across the living room, takes off her coat, and eases her down onto the couch.

DAVID

Don't go anywhere, sweetheart.

He walks into the kitchen and in a moment he is back with a tray that holds a newly-opened bottle of De Tierra Five-by-Five – their favorite wine – two crystal glasses, and a selection of nibbles. He puts it on the coffee table in front of her and sits down next to her. He pours two generous glasses, hands one to Lucy, and holds his own up to hers for a toast.

DAVID

To better days.

They clink glasses and take a sip of the wine.

LUCY

(Sighs) Better already.

DAVID

Miracle wine.

LUCY

David, you have spoiled me. Being with you these ten years, and especially over this last spell dealing with the virus, it has become all too clear that I am wasting my life.

DAVID

At the hospital? As a nurse?

She leans over and kisses him.

LUCY

Not specifically, my darling, just being anywhere that's not with you.

DAVID

I like that. Easy to fix. You have my full support. More. We can have a ceremony and burn your scrubs in the barbeque pit.

LUCY

And bury the ashes. (Sighs again, deeper, producing more relief. Shakes her head.) Today was the worst, and that's saying something. I haven't told you all that's been going on because I didn't want to worry you, but I'm done. That place is a disaster. The staff, the executives, and especially the patients.

DAVID

Lucy, I have wanted to make it up to you for the last two weeks. They were a fortnight of down-hills. I'll put you in full recovery mode. Please tell me what you need and when. Questions, answers, go for a walk, comfort food, favorite movies. My sole purpose is to restore you.

LUCY

Oh dear David, I feel that I've let you down,

falling so far.

DAVID

(Puts his arms around her, pulls her against him, rubs her back and neck) Silly girl, you have always given me more than I could ever have hoped for. And you're right. Being together is heaven, and we can have more of it...all of the time.

LUCY

(Tilts her head back, looks into his eyes.) I'm already feeling better.

DAVID

Oh, good. Maybe you can do your chores.

They both laugh.

DAVID

Sweetheart, would it help to tell me about today? What pushed you over the edge? And by the way, did you give notice?

LUCY

(Looking at him questioningly) Are you feeling your journalist oats?

DAVID

(Chuckles) Yes, I am. You've told me a lot about what's been happening at SMH, and I've seen a lot of stories online, mostly about other hospitals. Every day it gets worse, mostly because 97% of the Covid fatalities were people who didn't get vaccinated.

(Pauses, pours more wine) But I don't have to get on that horse now. I have a suggestion. Why don't you change out of your scrubs, put on some favorite soft togs, and we can go down to the beach?

LUCY

And maybe wind up at Dominic's for dinner?

DAVID

Ma certo. But of course.

LUCY

(Surprised look) I didn't know you learned Italian?

DAVID

Um, just a couple of useful phrases. Just for you because I always agree with you.

LUCY

(Frowns over a smile) Will you sign something that says that?

DAVID

Bien sûr, ma chère.

LUCY

What a good plan.

DAVID

(Pauses) Speaking of a plan, what do you think of my going undercover at the hospital to learn what I can first-hand and use the material to write a book?

LUCY

Or maybe a screenplay. No one reads books any-more. I know you could do a great script – plenty of blood and violence and corruption.

DAVID

(Laughs) That would fit in nicely with any primetime programming, wouldn't it?

LUCY

I'll get the popcorn. Oh, and I know a handful of people at the hospital who would love to help you. I will make a list of those I'm absolutely sure of in the different departments...people we can trust, and you can see who might fill any gaps.

DAVID

Good, but whatever you do, my darling, to help me with this, I don't want you to be the slightest bit vulnerable to any repercussions. I'll get any scrubs I need, if I do, at a costume shop. Nothing that can be traced to you.

LUCY

Not to worry, my love. Six hospitals all use the same laundry service for all the scrubs. There's no way they could be traced. And there are boxes full of identification badges of different shapes and colors no one knows what they actually refer to so not to worry. You tell me where you're going, and I'll outfit you.

DAVID

Grrrr. But I'll trust you.

LUCY

Good boy, and you can bake me a cake with a file in it if I wind up in the pokey.

DAVID

(Slow deep breath, smiling) How long are you going to stay there?

LUCY

Well, I have to give fair notice. First of all because they are so short-staffed, they don't have anyone that I've seen to fill in for me.

DAVID

I can't imagine they could replace you, even with two or three people.

LUCY

Why thank you, doctor, but you're still not going to get lucky with Lucy.

DAVID

(Chuckling) You have some considerable time coming to you, I think.

LUCY

Bunches. I have something like sixty sick days which I never took, and at least three months' vacation which I didn't take before I met you.

DAVID

I'll put a stop to that, my dear.

LUCY

Wonderfully, yes.

DAVID

That's serious bucks. Will they give you a hard time?

LUCY

I don't think so. The people in personnel know my numbers are right, and they know how much extra time I put in that I never put in for. Plus they would be nice hoping that they could persuade me to come back. Or fill in when there's a crunch.

DAVID

That's a good position to be in.

LUCY

Another good position would be lying on a beach somewhere. Maybe Cabo again. (Imagining) Oooh, yummy. Write your screenplay quickly, won't you?

DAVID

I could write it in a trice at Cabo, since I wouldn't have to worry about you at the hospital.

LUCY

I know what will put a bee in your proverbial bonnet. I'll give a one week notice and if you aren't mostly done with it, I'll stretch it another week.

DAVID

Oh judgment thou are fled to brutish beast, and this woman has lost her reason.

The Siren Ride

David is in the front seat of an ambulance, next to the driver, and the medic is in the back with two yet empty gurneys.

AMBULANCE DRIVER

(Driver to medic) Hey, Lopez, he's Nurse Lucy's guy. She asked us if he could ride along with us, to see what we gotta go through. All right with you?

AMBULANCE MEDIC

Yeah sure...anything for Nurse Lucy. She's great. (To David) I hope you've got a strong stomach. This can get pretty bad.

DAVID

Thanks for letting me ride along. I've been a journalist for a long time. I've seen a lot of bad stuff, including Vietnam. She told me you guys were the best.

AMBULANCE DRIVER

So like what are you looking for?

DAVID

(Deep breath, lets it out) The truth. I hear you fellows are working harder than you've ever had to before, what with this coronavirus, and the biggest problem is that the hospital isn't ready when you get there to take your patients.

The driver and medic looked at each other and then at David.

AMBULANCE DRIVER

Yeah, that's right. It's real bad.

AMBULANCE MEDIC

But you can't say it's just us. All the guys, they're getting the same thing.

DAVID

I've heard you've had to wait to come to the hospital because there are so many cases you can't even get near the ER entrance.

AMBULANCE MEDIC

(Nods his head, sadly and slowly) It was never like this before.

AMBULANCE DRIVER

No. We hear them calling in all the time. (nodding at the radio) They tell us to drive around for a while. Maybe try another hospital. It's no good. They're all filled up too.

DAVID

What are you supposed to do, just drive around?

AMBULANCE DRIVER

(Put his hands up in frustration) Like, what else can we do? And it's not their fault. The ER is full. They got cases in the hall, in the lobby they can't get to.

DAVID

(Quietly) Is there any form of triage?

AMBULANCE DRIVER

(Looks at his partner in the mirror who nods approval) There has to be. It's not like we call it that but that's what it is.

DAVID

What happens?

AMBULANCE DRIVER

There's a code. If the patient can still make it, he's a one. If it's not sure, he's a two.

DAVID

And if he's not going to make it...?

AMBULANCE MEDIC

Ain't gonna make, maybe even to the hospital, he's a three.

DAVID

(Whistles) Jesus. And that's in your hands? You have to make the determination?

AMBULANCE DRIVER

(Shakes his head) You know, if we've got a coupla threes like we did the other night, they tell us to jus' drive around, with the siren off. And when they're gone, we deliver them to the hospital morgue.

AMBULANCE MEDIC

(Clarifying) But their morgue's full most of the time now, with a lot of people who didn't make it in the ER, so they have us take 'em to the ice trucks.

AMBULANCE DRIVER

I know it sounds bad, but what can we do? I mean, there's always more calls. People who need us. And maybe we can help them on the scene, you know?

AMBULANCE MEDIC

They're a one or two.

AMBULANCE DRIVER

People at least who can make it. If we can get them into the hospital.

The ER

David is standing behind the desk of the ER Intake Manager, Rose Metafleur. They are separated by a heavy-duty plastic shield from the constant traffic of patients and staff coming and going to the Emergency Room.

DAVID

Lucy has sung your praises, Rose. She told me that you were a retired senior RN who had been called back into service when so many of your successors had burned out since the onset of the pandemic.

NURSE ROSE

(Shaking off the kudos) No one ever thought it would come to this. I read up on previous pandemics, here in the U.S. and elsewhere. I don't think we could have done anything fast enough to prepare, not after the idiot politicians dealing with the coronavirus from the beginning failed so miserably. They should have acted.

She is talking to David while she takes care of the continuing flood of paperwork from people on the other side of the plastic shield, and the incessant flashing alerts on her oversized computer screen. She somehow seems unfluttered.

NURSE ROSE

Especially Fauci and Birx...They knew how bad it was. They should have gone public with the truth instead of playing Trump toadies. Yeah, they would have been fired, but then they could have had a megaphone to tell the country what we needed to do to survive.

She scribbles a note and her initials on a form that is handed to her through a slit in the shield by a nurse who looked like she might fall down from exhaustion. Rose hands the form back to her. She turns quickly to see if David had seen what she had. He gives a quick nod.

NURSE ROSE

And she's not the worst of the bunch. I've been seeing faces like that for almost a year now. (Types instructions; two flashing alerts go away, leaving four) I mean, the U.S. has 4.25% of the world's population and 15% of the Covid deaths. You can't tell me it would have been that bad if those two "experts" had stood up to Trump. Plus the SOBs in the red states are blocking every safety measure – masks, spacing, vaccinations. Puhleeze. They should be charged with murder. At least negligent homicide.

A shattered young woman is standing on the other side of the plastic shield. She mumbles something Rose somehow understands.

NURSE ROSE

What's your father's name, hon?

When the woman is able to speak, she gives her a name. The name flies through Rose's fingers onto the screen. David sees her wince at the result.

NURSE ROSE

Yes, he's here. The doctors are working on him.

DAUGHTER

(Saw the wince, too) Can, can you tell me if he's going to be, you know, is he going to be alright?

NURSE ROSE

They'll do their best, hon. (Gives a demonstrable wince) It says here that he didn't think he'd had his shots.

DAUGHTER

(Shakes her head slowly) He said it wasn't safe.

NURSE ROSE

(In an even voice) Who told him that?

DAUGHTER

Someone on the TV. It was that Carlson person on Fox talking to someone. He was talking to an expert who said the vaccine had bad side effects which could be fatal.

NURSE ROSE

(To both the daughter and David) Yeah, I hear a lot of that. Hon, you can go for a walk if you want. I don't think there's any space in the waiting room. Hasn't been all night.

NURSE ROSE

(Touches a place on the computer screen and reads off a phone number) That's your mobile, isn't it? (Daughter nods.) We'll call you when he's out of the ER.

The daughter cringes as she realizes the two different ways he would come out. She turns around slowly, looks around at the chaos, and turns back to the woman behind the shield. She makes eye contact, nods slowly, says "Thank you" silently, and then walks toward the exit.

NURSE ROSE

(Shaking her head) They brought him in as a two, but they were being real generous. (Looks at David) It's the hardest part of the job to call a patient a three. (Shrugs) So only a few drivers do, so it's left to the triage doctor in charge of the ER. (Shows disgust) So many of them it's the same story. They don't get vaccinated for all the wrong reasons, and then they wait too late to call for help. (Caustic) The irony, of course, is that it makes our job easier. We don't really have a choice. Too many people coming through that door. We owe it to those who actually can pull through, to empty a bed for them to have their chance at surviving.

There is a flurry of activity for several minutes that Nurse Rose handles smoothly. Then there's something of a lull.

DAVID

How do the people in the ER handle this?

NURSE ROSE

(Looks at him for a long moment) Some of them don't.

DAVID

I can imagine.

NURSE ROSE

(Looks hard at him) No, you can't. Even if you were in there watching for a whole shift, you wouldn't know the feeling of deciding that someone is going to die. (Takes deep breath, lets it out) Of course, the purpose is to provide the medical attention to someone who is more likely to live. No one who hasn't had to make such a choice – here in the hospital or on the battlefield – can know what that does to a person, making such a decision. And no, you never get used to it. You never get numb to it. You succeed if it doesn't send you to the pharmacy. Which is often the final path. Then they have to find another. (Crosses her arms) You can take a look through the windows in the double doors to the ER, if you want. Not sure you can see much, or want to. The docs inside don't particularly like people looking in. I think you can understand that most people are clueless about what they are seeing. The other problem is that there have been a couple of times that people watched them working on a relative who didn't make it, and they found a shyster to sue the hospital and the doctors and everyone involved. No justification, of course, and the cases were thrown out of court. The defendants – our people – asked for legal fees and got 'em in a couple of cases. But you can understand why they are suspicious of spies. So they're rarely in the mood to have anyone looking in the window. (No response) You can try your luck. Don't know what you'll be able to see.

DAVID

Okay. Things seem to have quieted down some. I'll give it a try.

He walks out of the administration office and quietly proceeds to the ER doors. He stops, then sidles over for an angle view through a window. It isn't three minutes later that something large, red, and slimy strikes the window. It sticks momentarily and then slides off of the glass, leaving a bloody mess.

Nurse Rose has seen it from her desk. She can't hide her smile and keeps it until Skye returns to her office.

NURSE ROSE

If it's any consolation, that's happened on occasion to people who are inside the ER, instead of looking through the window.

DAVID

I'm counting my lucky stars, thank you.

The Dark Stars

David and Lucy are walking along a path by the river.

LUCY

I'm very glad that you are doing this book or screenplay, David, because it is important that people understand more about our health system, so they can make more informed choices about their own well-being.

DAVID

That's the key to all, isn't it? I mean coronavirus has upended a lot of how healthcare works in our society, but there's much of importance that has to be revealed and understood. You have already told me so much over the years, I have a good basic understanding of much of it, but I know that you have much more to tell me.

LUCY

You've been such a good listener, David. And

you got what I said so easily that it was exciting to tell you. I know it's because you're a journalist, but I've met a number in that field – I told you they had me fill in from time to time in the communications office when they needed someone to write an explainer for the public on something complicated – but none of them came close to holding a candle to you. It was the difference, as you once put it, between a job and a calling.

DAVID

I think that's why we got together so quickly and strongly, Lucy. Your commitment to your life-saving work and mine to life-informing.

LUCY

I hadn't thought about it that way, but you're right. Anyway, I love the way you listen and absorb. And ask the right questions that need answers. Your earnest listening mollified my more challenging experiences at SMH.

(Walking in silence) Especially the over-the-top tales of the biggest egos, the star doctors. You were really on target with that line you recalled from *Law and Order* when one of the cops said, "The difference between God and doctors is that God knows he's not a doctor." I didn't know whether to laugh or cry having seen such behavior so many times.

DAVID

That was a telling line.

LUCY

I've seen that attitude over the years, and I keep expecting – or hoping – that some of the young docs will get some humility. Don't know what it is. (Thinks) Maybe because they do actually save some lives, and they make living some lives better. And that's surely a big deal. But there are a lot of other folks, not doctors, who make peoples' lives better and they think that's being natural. You know, being kind. That can warm a lot of hearts.

DAVID

Tell me again, please, what you called your baptism by fire. I'd like it fresh in my mind.

LUCY

Ah yes. Well, I had been at the hospital only a few months and was working in the OR as a secondary nurse. My job was to support the primary nurses, which meant mostly disposing of used equipment and replacing supplies and tools. But I was fascinated by what went on in the OR so I was always watching everything closely. There was a critical moment when the surgeon was to inject a drug into the patient. I yelled "Stop!" The surgeon gave me a glance and was just about to insert the needle when I reached over and slapped his hand, knocking the hypodermic out of his hand. He was stunned and demanded, "What do you think you are doing?" Then he said, "She's fired. See that she's out of the building before I finish with this patient."

I didn't budge an inch. I said, "He picked up the wrong hypodermic. He would have killed the patient."

Suddenly everything stopped. Everyone was silent. All we heard were the machine sounds tracking of the patient's heart and lungs.

In a raised voice, the surgeon said, "I said get her out of here...Now!"

I bent over, picked up the hypodermic from the floor and walked out of the OR. I went up to the executive floor, and walked into the CEO's office without even knocking on his door. He was too shocked to protest. I said to him, "I've just been fired by Dr. Steinbrun. He was about to inject the patient with this." I held up the hypodermic. "I told him to stop. He ignored me and was about to inject the patient so I slapped it out of his hand. He was supposed to inject contrast dye but instead he'd received a syringe with a local anesthetic. It probably would have been fatal."

I stood there holding up the syringe. "Am I fired?"

The CEO looked back and forth from the syringe to me. "Uh, no. I don't think so."

"Thank you," I said and left his office. I went down to my locker and took a photograph of the hypodermic to record the digital identification that marked every shot to be delivered. Then I walked up to the lab and told one of the lab assistants, with whom I'd made friends, what had happened.

"Steinbrun is an egotistical bastard," she said. "I'm not surprised." She took the hypodermic from me and examined it, first by checking the digital number and then what was left in the syringe. "The number says it's Dilaudid, and I recognize the stuff by sight, touch, and smell. Yes, I can confirm that's what is in it." Then she leaned forward and gave me a kiss on the cheek. "Good job, girl. You probably saved the person's life."

DAVID

I do love the way you tell this story, my darling. Please tell me the rest.

LUCY

(Smiling) I never expected official acknowledgment from the hospital or humble appreciation from the doctor. For protection, during my lunch break I emailed the photograph and the lab confirmation to my attorney, explaining what happened. The attorney wasn't surprised. He knew all too well about doctors and hospitals. When I was back on duty, I was told by the head nurse that I was being reassigned to patient care. Which was actually something of an upgrade. And it was the work that I always wanted to do.

DAVID

Sweetheart, I remember when you first told me about it. We'd been together only a short time. You said giving you the assignment you wanted, taking care of patients who needed you, was sort of hush money.

LUCY

(Laughed, walked closer to him) Yes, and it was what made it possible for me to meet you, my wonderful man.

DAVID

(In a faux rough tone) Lucy, back to work.

LUCY

(Laughing) Yessir, Doctor.

DAVID

How has the pandemic changed the behavior of the doctors?

LUCY

Hmm, good question. I'd like to say that it has humbled them – it should have – but I haven't seen a lot of that. Maybe those who aren't working on Covid patients are a little less pushy, aware of how much those colleagues are going through. Most of them are simply exhausted. (Thinking) I wonder if they will change back when it's over. If it's ever over.

DAVID

The people you work with whom I've met and seen since Covid hit, they don't seem as sure of themselves. I wonder if it's about their profession, their own job, or what is happening in the world today.

LUCY

I wish I could say it's about the world today, but I don't see that. I don't hear it in the conversations. I don't see any change in how they treat their patients.

DAVID

Wow, and you see it up close and personal. They spend a couple of minutes with the patients, but you spend far more time with them. Where do you suppose they got this attitude toward life? The god–ish importance that limits what they can see or care about?

LUCY

(Frowning) I don't know. But here's a clue. When they save a patient's life, or just take care of a problem that gives them a better life, they appear more proud about their professional success than about the patient doing well. Not all of them, of course, but a good number of them.

DAVID

(Shaking his head) And if the patient dies, or the operation that would have produced happier days doesn't produce the hoped-for results, has the doctor failed or was it the patient's fault.

LUCY

Oh, I think you could answer that from what you've learned over the years and heard from me. It may have been the patient not doing what he was supposed to, or not making enough of an effort. Or something might have gone askew in the diagnosis by an earlier doctor. Or the disease was just too advanced. Dot-dot-dot.

DAVID

But it was never the doctor's fault. He did his best.

LUCY

Yes. He's always done his best.

Family Matters

David has just come into the house after getting the mail. He shuffles through the envelopes and stops when he sees one of particular interest. He continues rifling through the rest, and then drops all but the one on the table and opens it. He finds a card with little writing on it and reports to Lucy who is sitting on the couch.

DAVID

I sent the invite to Phyllis Clavell for dinner. (He holds up the card) She responded. She said Phyllis and Wiff will be delighted to attend. I guess she meant to write "wife."

LUCY

(Smiling but not resolving his confusion) You didn't know that she preferred females?

DAVID

It never came up, so to say.

LUCY

(Laughing hard) Darling, Phyllis meant to write Wiff. That's her dog. (Laughs more) A bitch, I should note. Phyllis has always had a dog. And always a female. That part I don't know why. Oh, and she brings Wiff with her wherever she goes, except to the hospital. She doesn't want her to come down with something from there.

DAVID

(Chuckles) Very funny. I like that. So I'll get to meet them both on Saturday night. From the way you described her, she sounds grand.

LUCY

I know you'll like them both.

*   *   *   *   *

It's Saturday night. The three humans are sitting at the dinner table. Wiff is lying curled up on a nearby rug. Having finished what was obviously a very sating meal, they are enjoying cordials.

PHYLLIS

Yeah, I get it. Time to sing for my supper, as it were.

DAVID

Lucy explained to you what this is all about.

Gathering information for a book or screenplay on what it's like in hospitals under the pandemic siege.

PHYLLIS

It sure ain't *Dr. Kildare* if it ever was, and when Lucy told me I thought what you're doing is a good idea. People need to understand how much more difficult – awful – it is for everyone. The doctors and nurses, the patients and their families. We'd all be better off if people understood what we're all dealing with – problems we haven't had to face before. Especially the crowds and the long days. And so many dying. So I'm here for you. What can I tell you?

DAVID

Again, thank you for coming Phyllis. And thank you for bringing Wiff. I'm ever more inclined to have such a wonderful creature in our home.

PHYLLIS

(Winks at Lucy) Looks like you got a smart one, my friend.

LUCY

(Smiles; soft voice) I couldn't have done better.

DAVID

(Smiles back at her) Thank goodness that shot

sent me into the hospital. (Shakes his head) Anyway, Phyllis, please tell me your background. (Starts a micro recorder sitting on the table between them)

PHYLLIS

For the longest time I've been a traveling nurse. I did stints in hospitals around the country for usually three months, sometimes longer, and then moved on to another facility, usually in another city and often in another state.

DAVID

I think when I met you a couple of years ago you were at Santa Marino for a short while. And if I remember, you'd already been on the road for some 30 years and had set up shop in more than sixty locations, a number of them like Santa Marino, more than once.

PHYLLIS

That's right, and I think I did another score of hospitals since then.

DAVID

You're handling the intake at SMH now. Is this going to be temporary or are you headed off to somewhere else soon.

PHYLLIS

(Sighs) I never know. I love the area but the workload is grueling. I'm not sure it wouldn't be elsewhere, or if this place might lighten up. It couldn't get worse. I guess it all depends on the virus.

LUCY

Phyllis has one of the hardest jobs in nursing and that's dealing with the families. It was before the pandemic, certainly during it, and it won't change at least until the pandemic ends, if it ever does.

PHYLLIS

It's stunning, and tragic, how little people know about human beings and what it takes to keep them healthy. And that's everywhere. I've been everywhere, almost. From frosty New England to the Deep South, from the Black Hills in South Dakota to the glitter of Hollyweed. And that means I've talked to a lot of people. Sometimes the families are effective conduits to getting the patients to really understand what they and we are dealing with. They can get through better than me. But so many of them, particularly members of the same family, have been living similar toxic lives; smoking, drinking too much, maybe doing drugs. Or they're punishing the scale at 300 pounds. Plus they're loud, which suggests they don't listen, or are absolutely silent which is almost as bad since you can't get the information you need from them.

LUCY

It must be a challenge with so many varied types of family relationships.

PHYLLIS

Oh my goodness, it can be crazy. Even before Covid when family could be in the patients' room. Crazy on top of the critical situation of the patient, medical needs, doctors and nurses popping in. That, all on top of the various relationships with the patient and among themselves.

DAVID

People used to behave better not so long ago. There was dignity and compassion.

PHYLLIS

(Chuckles) I remember those days. I trace it back to when the churches allowed people to come in flip-flops and shorts. To keep the coffers filled, of course, but they lost the solemnity in the process.

LUCY

This is slightly off track – and this is not just Covid but there's more of it now – but one of the things that gets me about the people coming to say their last goodbyes is that they kept encouraging the patient to fight whatever it is that's killing him. Fight he might, of course, but it isn't going to do any good. The patient is fighting just to make the family feel better even though he is actually ready to leave.

PHYLLIS

And all too often already in considerable pain.

LUCY

Yes. I don't understand why the family doesn't understand that. And let him pass.

PHYLLIS

(Raised her eyebrows) Isn't it because we don't understand death? That's certainly the way most people in our country, and much of Western culture act. If people understood what was happening, physically and emotionally, they would honor the needs of the patient. Instead they are selfish. More out of ignorance than anything else.

DAVID

Phyllis, has it been any different with the coronavirus?

PHYLLIS

Yes, it has. Like everything else. And in a number of ways. I mean first, so many of the patients are dying. Second, most of the visitors can't get near the patient, even if they've been vaccinated. Another difference is that we encounter a lot more belligerence from the families. Some of them insist that Covid is a hoax.

DAVID

Of course, they haven't been vaccinated.

PHYLLIS

Not them, not the patient, though I can't tell you how many of the people who are sick with the virus ask to be vaccinated. Of course it's too late; they can't be. The family especially doesn't want to hear "no" and they are known to get violent with the hospital staff, saying things like, "Give me a shot and let me see her." (Shakes her head in disgust and dismay) Again, it's all about them. Their rights and taking no responsibility.

DAVID

It sounds like you have little sympathy for these people, the family.

PHYLLIS

Yes, David, I guess that's true. Not only are so

many of them crass and often difficult to control per the needs of the hospital, most haven't been vaccinated. They don't get in. Plus, as you probably have guessed, we're seeing a lot of fake vaccination cards. We have screening devices that catch most of them.

DAVID

What do you do with them?

PHYLLIS

No f-ing around. We confiscate them. And if they object, we hand them over to the police. Yeah, the police. We have one or two at the main door the visitors come through, and they don't like this nonsense any more than we do. These cretins will be charged with a misdemeanor. It won't mean jail time, but the worse they complain, the bigger the fine. The night court judges are very much on our side, because the perps are such obvious imbeciles and they whine and shout.

DAVID

Judging from what I've seen when I'm picking up Lucy, you have considerably more security.

PHYLLIS

Oh yes. We started with twice the normal contingent of private cops, but quickly found we needed more. Also, we had to install more sophisticated locks. All but the main doors where I am are one-way out. And the staff, including the doctors, are all admitted through face or palm recognition screens. Teehee to them...they thought they shouldn't even have to show ID.

LUCY

(Quick look at David; asks Phyllis) Do people try to come in wearing scrubs?

PHYLLIS

(Laughs) Yes, but their ideas of what they should look like they get from television. Not quite *Ben Casey*. More like *St. Elsewhere* or *House* but still obvious.

LUCY

What happens to them?

PHYLLIS

The police register their real IDs and then we stamp an indelible "Fake" in unmissable places on their clothes. Hah. They won't be able to return them to costume rental store.

They sit silently for a couple of minutes, with no sense of urgency to talk. Then Phyllis sighs deeply and her demeanor softens dramatically.

PHYLLIS

But it's so sad when the people are truly loving and close to the patient. Their wanting to get close, to touch, to kiss goodbye is genuine. It's not protocol for them, its real feelings, and you can see that it goes both ways. But they can't get near them, usually not in the same room, only looking through a window and from a distance. There's a lot of crying. A real sadness. As you'd expect from real people. I sometimes think they would be better off not saying goodbye in person, maybe on the phone. (Eyes moist; sniffs; clears to a smile) But there have been some good times too. When they get to the hospital and the person has taken a turn toward recovery. It's rare. I mean, the doctors hold off on a death sentence as long as possible, so it rarely reverses, but sometimes it does. Then everyone is ecstatic as you can imagine. (Chuckles) We had someone rent one of those 100-foot tree-cutter devices – super cherry pickers – and they brought the bucket up close to the third-floor window where the patient was so they could say goodbye. The cops weren't terribly happy about it but when the husband and daughter were brought down after a few minutes, the girl sobbing, they let them go. Also the guy with the truck. He knew the patient, too, and he was as much a mess, not even going up to see her, as was her family.

LUCY

Amazing...tragic too, that so much of your time and resources is diverted just to keep order.

PHYLLIS

Yes. And no one has a sense that it's gonna end anytime soon. Even after the Covid threat is gone. Maybe when enough people die that whoever is left will wake up and get their shots. But what we've seen so far, it's hard to even hope for that.

Phyllis gets up from her chair. As do Lucy and David.

PHYLLIS

Time to go. Wiff and I are passionate about watching *The Three Stooges* and they're on at eleven. We watch every night, instead of the news.

LUCY

(Goes into the kitchen and returns with a bag she had fixed) Some leftovers for you and some bones for Wiff.

DAVID

Thank you, Phyllis, for what you told us, and for

what you've done for all these years. Please stay healthy.

PHYLLIS

Glad I could contribute in my own small way, you two. Let us know if there is anything else you need.

The Splintered Board

David is sitting at his desk reading the *Santa Marino Star* on his computer when Lucy, wearing her running togs, comes in with the coffee pot to refill his cup.

DAVID

Thank you, gorgeous. (Shakes his head) It amazes me how you look so beautiful every time I look at you.

LUCY

(Kisses him on the cheek) It's your charming way of saying thank you for the table service.

DAVID

That may be the case, but it's also true. (Taps some keys, pulls up what's in his email inbox, and points at one of the listings) What's that look like to you?

LUCY

(Reads) LoveYourLucy@gmail.com. What's that?

DAVID

I was hesitant to open it. It also has a good size video file. But the more I thought about it, the more it seemed friendly.

LUCY

(Humorously) You mean no nasty pictures of your girlfriend?

David puts his hand behind her neck and gently brings her lips down to his for a long kiss. He slowly lets go.

DAVID

(Strong but quiet voice) I've had girlfriends, Lucy. You've heard about some of them. You, my dear, are not my girlfriend. (Pauses) You are my life.

Lucy leans down for another long kiss.

LUCY

(In a husky voice) You are still very charming. (Points to the email; clears her throat) And I think you should open it. It feels friendly to me, too.

DAVID

(Nods) But I'll send it to the other computer to open it.

LUCY

I think it's very clever of you to have kept that old machine, David, to check out suspicious files. If there's anything wrong, you won't risk all you've got on this one.

David clicks some keys and watches the email appear on the old computer. He opens it and starts the video.

DAVID

(Smiles) Oh my goodness, this is a video of last night's hospital board room.

LUCY

(Broad smile) Ha! I bet we know who sent that. That would be Jake Olander, the person in charge of the hospital's A/V operations. I introduced you to him a while back. Some hospital affair. A very good fellow. His wife is wonderful too.

DAVID

Yes. Good guy. (Frowns) I didn't know that they were videotaping the board of directors meetings. Did you?

LUCY

(Shakes her head; thinks) But you must have impressed him, David, that he thought to send it to you. It must be significant.

DAVID

It doesn't surprise me that they video'd the meetings as a reasonable record-keeping practice for years. Then there wasn't a need for the secretary to keep notes. That made sense back in the days when the hospital saw itself as a major player in the community's health and healing.

LUCY

I wish that they had stayed that course. I wonder if they forgot that they were being recorded...when the directors were more focused on how the hospital could be "more efficient."

DAVID

And show higher figures in the profit column.

LUCY

(Sighs) Yes. (Remembers) Jake told me that he had set up the cameras and microphones carefully so that they covered everyone in the boardroom but were virtually invisible. At least out of casual sight.

DAVID

My guess is then that it wasn't too long before the members forgot about them, or at least stopped expressing interest in seeing the recordings. That would make sense since there would be a certain cockiness about the power of the group. Especially after they replaced three members who weren't quite so on the same page with the others about the importance of reaching financial goals. After that, why would anyone want to see the recordings?

LUCY

Maybe not the board, but maybe if someone was concerned about one of them having said something that wouldn't look good to outsiders. I mean, there were plenty of issues with the pandemic moving into full swing. The stress level had to grow and there had to be fewer unanimous votes.

DAVID

(Chuckled) Yeah, particularly about how much they should pocket and what risks were worth taking.

LUCY

Honey, I really have to run and feel if I don't do it now, I'll just sloth the rest of the day. I know you ran earlier. I don't imagine you want to take another one? (Sees his no) Can you wait to watch the video so I can watch it with you?

DAVID

Of course. Yes, I had a good run while you were still sleeping. Take your time. I'd rather watch it with you anyway. You know about some of the board members and will be able to fill in some holes for me.

Lucy kisses him on his proffered cheek and walks out of his office. He hears her leave through the back door.

David makes good use of the time, brewing a fresh pot of coffee and cutting up several pastries. Soon after he is done, he hears her footsteps on the back deck. He opens the door for her and she double-takes on some crumbs on his face.

LUCY

Someone ate the canary. (Leans toward him; licks some crumbs from his face) Mmm. You're delicious. (Laughs) I'll shower quick and meet you in your office in ten minutes.

DAVID

Don't rush, sweetheart. Enjoy the steam.

David works at his computer for a few minutes and

then goes to the kitchen where he puts the coffee, cups, and treats on a tray, carries it into his office and places it on a table away from his work area. Lucy appears, looking relaxed. They make themselves comfortable and David rolls the video.

The first shot is a message from Olander saying that he has sent the pertinent clips from what was originally a two-hour meeting. In what he has sent, they will see the twelve people around the board table, two of them women; one woman and two of the men are the commanding voices of the meeting. It is all tightly run. There are five agenda items to be discussed and three of the issues reveal some disagreement. At the end, as the members got up and left, several of the faces made it clear that the dissenters had not been mollified. Then it was over.

LUCY

It wasn't always like that, David. I went to a few board meetings in the first years I was there. For one thing, more of the members participated. Also, the proposals were modified as a result.

DAVID

None of the rubber-stamping we saw happening last night.

LUCY

The vice chair – what did you call her, The

Dragon Woman? – doesn't seem to have had the slightest interest in negotiating. That's not healthy. And those wanting to tweak the proposals the way they were presented actually made some sense.

DAVID

No. Judging by what I saw on their faces, that's why the chair put her in that position. He wouldn't have to take the heat.

LUCY

(Shakes her head) So what do you think? Anything to be done with it? Jake sure thought so to send it to you.

DAVID

Well the three issues that caught my attention, and raised some hackles, were how they were negotiating with the insurance companies, requiring vaccinations or testing for the ambulance workers, security workers, and contract staff, and accepting religious exemptions.

LUCY

(Intrigued) Yes, I agree. Those were the biggies. What is your take on them? Why are they important? And what would you do differently about them?

DAVID

(Straight-faced) Take a breath, will ya? Are you running for the vice's seat?

LUCY

(Laughs) Oh, David, I can just imagine what a much better job the hospital – the people at the hospital could be doing – if they had righteous management.

DAVID

(Nodding) More coffee, Lucy, or maybe a drink?

LUCY

No, David, I'm good. Sometimes I lose patience with the people making the decisions in our world.

DAVID

Yes, but you are so gracious about it. I think they should all be imprisoned.

LUCY

I could go that way.

DAVID

I was doing a podcast the other day with Rebecca, and doing the right thing came up. We talked about how hospitals, colleges and universities, and news operations all used to be about serving the needs of the people. And now they are just going after the buck. I said, just imagine what a valuable tool Facebook – or Meta as they're calling it – could be if it did things right. They'd probably make even more money, while they were serving our information-hungry planet.

LUCY

Yes, but how do we get there, David?

DAVID

My dearest, Zuckerberg is not on my speed dialer. But I have some thoughts about how to bring some appropriate attention to the issues before the SMH board. Not that they'll snap to, but the tactical point I want to make is that they are always leaning forward, ready to defend, argue, and refuse to retreat. What they first need to do is get them off balance and then give them an alternative path to move them to a better place than where they were headed.

LUCY

Why David, it sounds so simple but it's truly brilliant. Not that I'm surprised. Any details?

DAVID

Well, first of all, my most value partner in everything, it was your comment about imagine the SMH doing the right thing. That was the key. Thank you.

LUCY

(Blushing above a broad smile) Why thank you, my love. Should I open a bottle of something to get things flowing?

DAVID

There's a bottle of La Marca in the fridge and a couple of appropriate glasses in the freezer.

LUCY

Prosecco. Perfect.

She gets up, leans over to deliver a sloppy kiss to David, and heads to the kitchen.

DAVID

Hey, Miss Tease, ya know, we could do the heavy thinking later.

LUCY

(From the kitchen) Nah, You're much too easily distracted. The bubbly will help you focus.

DAVID

(Chuckles) Uh-huh.

Lucy returns with the Proseco and the glasses. David

opens the bottle and pours liberal amounts. They clink their glasses and take a good sip.

DAVID

All right, the big factor for them with these three issues – dealing with the insurance companies, vaccinating the worker bees, and exempting religious exemptions – is public relations, at least the last two. Let's start with the religious exemptions.

There is a montage of shots of David explaining, Lucy asking questions, David responding, along with their looking at parts of the video again. David finishes his take on how the board might shift and get further ahead with different approaches.

LUCY

Oh that's excellent. It makes so much sense. Dollars and cents.

She fills both glasses and holds hers up to his for a toast and a big sip.

DAVID

So I know who the vice is, I've met the chief – Abel Wormser – several times at the SMH chichi cocktail parties. Seems like a good guy, considering. I'm not sure he should be approached directly. What are your thoughts, my dear, and who is that third guy who had a lot to say?

LUCY

Jerome Satay. I think you've met him. You talked briefly. Big bucks investor, he has important connections in the medical equipment world.

DAVID

Hmm. Yes, I met him. I was talking with him when he had to take a call. I didn't wait around. (Thinks) I wonder if he might not be the entry point. Judging from what he said on those three issues, he wasn't overjoyed at the direction Wormser was letting things go.

LUCY

I was impressed by him. He listens to people, as long as they are saying something intelligent. I didn't talk with him, but I watched him. Discerning fellow. David, he would listen to you.

DAVID

Is he local?

LUCY

From what I read, he has four or five homes around the world in major hotels. He loves being by the ocean. I think he stays at the Coronado when he's in this corner of the world. And I think they give him a nice office at the hospital when he's in town. He's a serious hands-on board member.

DAVID

Please see if you can find out when he will be in his office, if that's possible.

LUCY

Will do. But not, I think, until we finish the La Marca. I put another bottle in the freezer.

Without the Nurses

David and Lucy are in the kitchen making dinner.

DAVID

Do you think you might get a few nurses to talk about their hospital experiences under Covid?

LUCY

(Thinks) Yes, I should be able to do that. But I think they would be more willing to talk if they were alone with me.

DAVID

That's fine. Better that they are unreserved.

LUCY

And we promised to not use any names.

DAVID

Sure. Dunno if this would grease the wheels but I could rent a private room at one of the local restaurants and buy them all lunch or dinner.

LUCY

(Hopeful look) Would you buy my lunch or dinner, too?

DAVID

Well, okay, but no alcohol for you.

LUCY

(Laughs) Oh, dang, to use your favorite word.

DAVID

They should be willing for you to record the conversation so that you don't have to take notes. And once it is transcribed by an Internet AI program, the recording will be erased.

LUCY

They'll like that. Good.

*　　　*　　　*　　　*　　　*

There are three women and one man, and they are actually anxious to talk about their experiences under the pandemic conditions. They have coordinated their schedules so that they could meet the next Sunday at eleven, two of them attending early mass to accommodate the others. That day and that hour made it easy for Lucy to find a room at a nice restaurant not in the immediate area. She didn't have to tell her colleagues to come in civvies. On the table are small flower bouquets from David for all five nurses. Lucy hadn't known about them. They sit down, read the menu, order their food, and then get down to business.

LUCY

Thank you again, all of you, each of you, for coming here this morning. I know it's a new thing for you, but I know that when it's done, and you see the results, you will be very proud to have participated. All of us have been working at SMH, and many of us at other hospitals, too, and we've seen a lot and seen a lot that could be done better. That's what this is all about.

*   *   *   *   *

When Lucy arrives home that afternoon, her eyes are red. David wraps his arms around her and holds her tight, massaging her back and neck.

DAVID

Oh, sweetheart, I'm sorry. How thoughtless of me to put you through the pain.

Lucy relishes the rubbing for a good couple of minutes before she pulls her head back.

LUCY

You'll do more of that later, won't you?

He squeezes her as a reply. She returns her head to his chest briefly and then pulls away.

LUCY

I should have known that it would affect me, David. I mean, I know a lot of the chaos and the brutality, but many of the details were new, and awful.

She takes a microcassette from her pocket and hands it to him.

LUCY

You can listen to it, if you want, I trust you. So would they. Or you can just get the transcription made. My guess is that you will want to get to work right away. It is that compelling.

DAVID

(Nods) It'll likely be a couple of hours, and then we can go for a long walk by the ocean. (Kisses her; kisses her again.)

David has set up for recording a top to this section. He moves closer to the microphone and records his intro.

DAVID

Many doctors see nurses as the people who follow the elephants in the parade, cleaning up their messes. Not the good doctors, of course.

They know that their patients would have a far worse time of their hospital stay if it weren't for the personal concern and professional attention of the nurses. But during the best of times, a heavy load is put on their shoulders. During the pandemic, it has been hell. We spoke with four nurses who had been working for years before the coronavirus struck and have been working through it. Here's what they had to say.

David stops his recording and uploads the audio from the microcassette to his computer. He inserts the nurses' recording behind his intro and then uploads the package to a site that will transcribe it. The site will fill in the five names that David then feeds them. While it is producing the transcript, he listens to the nurses' recording that brought Lucy home in tears.

ANN

We're not just taking care of their medical needs. The worst thing is we're filling in for their families who can't be there, when they need family the most. The people they love and who may never hold them again. How do you fill that role?

BETTY

We're dealing with people who are never going to leave the hospital. They only leave the bed they're in when they die. How do you comfort them? What can you possibly say? Early on, we might gently ask them why they didn't get vaccinated, but now, what's the point? It doesn't matter what the reason was. They didn't. They're going to die because they made this fatal mistake. And there's nothing we can do or say that can make up for what they didn't do.

CAROL

It's harder for us, you know. It's gotta be. I mean, the doctors, especially those in the ER, they usually see the patient once. But we see the patients from beginning to end. And the end is often their last breath. (Sobs, sniffs) Here's something for you. That last breath. For the patient and the nurse it means the end. For the patient, the pain is over but not for us.

ANN

One thing I don't understand is that only 25% of pregnant women are getting vaccinated. And that's what it has climbed to. I don't know if they are honestly afraid that it will hurt their fetus or they're just using it as an excuse. In any event, I find it deplorable that a would-be mother would put her newborn at risk. What kind of mother is she going to be? And imagine how the child will be crippled when she inevitably learns that her mother needlessly died to protect her baby. I mean, science shows that babies are born better protected if the mother has been vaccinated.

DOUG

What gets me is the never-ending nature of this. There's really an almost overwhelming sense of hopelessness. I mean, when's the next variant coming and what will it be? It's hard to imagine that it could be worse, but we thought we'd had seen the worst and then Delta came along. We know that viruses mutate, making themselves less vulnerable to medicines. What will the next variant be?

CAROL

That's what scares me. People ask, when will this all be over, and we don't know. We don't know if it ever will be...in our lifetimes...either.

ANN

What gets me most is that the people who are the most angry are the anti-vaxxers, or at least the people who just haven't gotten their shots. Who are they to talk? And why should they put their anger on us? They are the ones who are brewing up the next batch of death. But they're so blind to the truth. There's nothing you can say to them.

DOUG

I don't understand why the government doesn't step in and stop lies and misinformation. They should shut down those right-wing television and radio stations that deny there's a virus and tell people they don't need to be vaccinated or wear masks.

BETTY

The worst is the social media. They put out all the false stuff like ivermectin to take for Covid. We had two people in here last month who had overdosed on that stuff. And before, remember, chloroquine and hydroxychloroquine; Trump was promoting that, and some people were drinking bleach. How could people be so stupid? I sometimes think that we should refuse to treat people who do that.

DOUG

Sometimes I think we shouldn't have to treat anyone who hasn't been vaccinated. Their insurance companies shouldn't cover them either. I mean, 95-some percent of the Covid patients here, and across the country, didn't get their shots. That's why they are here, filling up our beds unnecessarily. And they're taking up beds from people who have all sorts of problems that weren't their fault, like cardio, accidents, cancer.

ANN

All these years, I've wondered about the people who are taking up space because they smoke cigarettes, drank too much alcohol, or did drugs. These people are responsible for being here. Why should other people who were trying to stay healthy be paying for them?

CAROL

Or the people who are obese? How did more than 40% of American adults put on a hundred extra pounds or more? And it made them three times more susceptible to the coronavirus. You're right, why can't we hold people responsible? (Clears her throat) I don't really mean that. (Adds) Not all the time.

BETTY

I don't disagree with you. (Chuckles) Not all the time. But they not only fill up our beds, but they create so much extra work, for the doctors, for us, and the people who are changing the linens and loading the oxygen tanks. They are bleeding the energy out of us. It's gotten so I don't feel like we are really making a difference. I mean, I know that's not true, but I don't have the time to give our patients the attention they need.

ANN

That's what gets me the most. I used to see every patient like I wasn't in a hurry. Now I check their numbers and that's about it. I don't have time to even ask how they are feeling. That's not nursing, not what I signed up for.

BETTY

Signed up for is right. I have to tell you, as much I appreciate working with all of you, and some of the doctors and staff, I think about quitting. Maybe not quit nursing, but leaving the hospital. Go into travel nursing. I have a nice home but I don't have any family here. And those travel nurses are getting four or five times what I'm getting here.

CAROL

I've thought about that too. My kids are gone. I don't have to see my ex ever again. And the money would be nice. Plus some places, they are putting nurses up in nice apartments or hotels. And I have to think that going to new places, instead of being fed up with the same-ole, um, stuff, we have here, I'd have time to figure out the differences at the new place. They would cut me slack 'cause I was new and not give me a hard time. And anyway, it would be easier knowing that I could be gone from wherever in a couple of months.

DOUG

That may be an answer. I confess that I was thinking of leaving the hospital and finding a group practice where there wasn't the chaos and abuse. Or just find a new kind of work. Maybe be an influencer.

(Laughter)

CAROL

What would you influence about?

DOUG

How 'bout a campaign to vote only for people who supported vaccinations?

ANN/BETTY/CAROL

Yes. Agreed. I'll contribute.

(Silence)

ANN

It has to get better...some time. Two years ago, I was caring for five patients on a shift. Now on nights, I've got ten, even more. That's crazy. It can't last. Or I can't.

BETTY

I saw an article the other day about a study that

spoke of moral distress. It can get so discouraging that people start thinking about suicide. I mean, it's so upsetting, with no change in sight, that they – nurses were the topic – just don't see a way out.

CAROL

You haven't reached that stage, have you?

BETTY

No. That was in the article. And thank goodness I have you, my friends. You are so much more than colleagues.

ANN

You can call me anytime, all of you. Know that. Not that I'm stronger, but especially over the past 18 months or however long it has been, you have become like family to me. (Sniffs)

DOUG

You are my sisters. I know guys aren't good for anything but killing spiders and lifting heavy boxes, but I am always here for you.

ANN

Thank you, Doug.

BETTY

I'm with you.

CAROL

I've got some heavy boxes in my garage that need moving. (Laughter) You know, talking about family, because so few families are permitted to see the patients, even those who don't have Covid, but they are trying to keep everyone safe, I feel a need to fill in the gap, especially with the women in the labor room. The first-timers who are just having their baby. No Covid. Nothing else. They are very needy, oh my god, and they should be. Not always frightened but desperate for someone who knows what they are going through. I don't resent them being seriously needy because I had three children myself and I know how important it was to have family around. I mean, maybe it's not a big deal when you've had a whole bunch of kids, but my mother was with me when I delivered, and my husband and sister spent lots of time with me in the three days I was in the hospital. That meant everything to me.

DOUG

I think giving that compassionate attention is the most important part of the job. At least it is for me. Not as a job, but as a human being. And with the pandemic and all the beds filled, I feel I'm not able to give everything I have. That's why I resent the people who shouldn't be taking up beds because they wouldn't get vaccinated. They are not only stupid and selfish, and putting other people in jeopardy, but they are taking precious attention that I want to give to people who truly need and deserve it.

ANN

If you do go off and become an influencer, I want you to rant and rave against the governors who have banned regulations mandating vaccination and even requiring masks and social distancing. Those states have the lowest vaccination stats.

DOUG

And the most overflowing hospital facilities.

ANN

How can they be so, so...what is it? It can't just be stupid, if they managed to get elected. Are they afraid they won't get re-elected? Or are they evil? I don't understand.

DOUG

There is blood on their hands. The blood of thousands of people.

BETTY

But it's not just the governors and state legislators. It's the people of those states. Many of them must support their governors, foolishly or ignorantly. But I think it was something said before, about the misinformation that people are buying into. There was a story I saw that somewhere in the Midwest, people were being told that they wouldn't be permitted to carry a concealed gun if they were wearing a mask. Carrying a gun was so important to them that they wouldn't wear a mask? How crazy is that?

CAROL

Please God. End this insanity. Let us have our lives back so that we can do your work.

*   *   *   *   *

DAVID

That should shake the wheels off the carriage. Hearing it was one thing. It would be grand if every doubter could listen to them. The voices packed with so much meaning, so much emotion. But reading the words, with a little punctuation, you can certainly get most of the power and the pain.

David hands Lucy the transcript he's printed out for her. She sits down on the couch with her tea and reads through it. When she is done, her eyes are red again.

LUCY

It didn't lose much, David. I think ending it with the comment about how crazy are the deniers. That will give you a good lead into the issue of the people who are refusing to get vaccinated...Are they insane, literally?

DAVID

That's right. Do you have anything you want to add that wasn't covered in the interview?

LUCY

A couple of things, actually. One that Betty brought up after. She is an ardent follower of the HIPAA regulations on privacy, and she said she was further frustrated by not being able to tell her husband about what she was dealing with. Just being able to talk to other nurses gave her some release, but she wanted to explain what she was going through to her husband and her older children so they would understand her moods. She has to stuff so much inside herself. Another point is about the whole hospital situation, not just nurses though it certainly makes our job much more difficult, and that is the overcrowding. Average patient stays were about four to five days, but the serious Covid patients will stay more than two weeks, and while it might seem counterintuitive, the research shows that the longer they are in the hospital, the worse it will mean for them. For us it also means that we don't have anywhere near the rooms or enough beds. We have patients in hallways, the lounges in the upper floors, even in storage closets. That's bad enough, but it means that we don't have anywhere to put the people coming out of the ER, which means we can't make space for the new patients, who are most in need of emergency care. Not just Covid but accident victims whose lives depend on medical intervention in minutes. And you can't provide that kind of care in the lobby. The equipment that saves lives is in the ER. We can also run low on supplies, especially with what's happened to delivery schedules, for our needs as well as everyone else's.

DAVID

I hate to ask, Lucy, if there's anything more because I know there is, and it seems overwhelming.

LUCY

It is overwhelming. Overwhelming and insane. Or because so many people are acting insane, it has become overwhelming. People seem to think that Covid is only taking down the seniors, who they imagine are the chronically sick, and which many of the younger people think of as anyone over fifty. But in fact, we've been seeing people our own age and younger; people in their twenties. These are the age of their children, for goodness sakes. (Takes a deep breath; lets it out) And one more thing. I don't think we've seen a single new patient who wasn't in denial about having the virus, mostly because they somehow were trying to justify to themselves why they didn't get vaccinated, who refused to seek hospital care until it was too late, for most of them. Had they come in after a day or two, we might have helped them. After five days or a week, they weren't going to leave alive.

DAVID

(Pulls her against him) It was shortly after we met, after that insane PR stunt with the guns, that I told you I didn't see how the world could get itself back on the rails until there was a disease based on consciousness. One that would take out those at the lower end of the spectrum and give those of us in the higher reaches of awareness, compassion, and intellect the opportunity to truly realize the potential of caring hearts and bright minds.

LUCY

Yes, I do remember that conversation, my darling man. I thought it was the best path that our species could take. (Eyes widen) Goodness gracious, David, do you think that's what's happening?

DAVID

Considering who's not getting vaccinated, it certainly fits the bill.

Sri Satay

Lucy is calling David on her cellphone from the hospital.

LUCY

David, Jerome Satay's secretary is out for the morning. He's in his office, I think enjoying some quiet time to get some work done without being disturbed.

DAVID

Terrific, sweetheart. Thank you. Great timing. I just finished doing some research on him. His parents were from Ceylon. That was before the island's name was changed back to its original name in 1972. He was born in Palo Alto, went to Stanford and then the London School of Economics. His success as an investor is almost exclusively in companies that are socially beneficial and has driven his wealth close to ten figures.

LUCY

(Laughs) Go get him, my tiger.

*   *   *   *   *

David walks past the empty desk of his secretary and through the door into Satay's office

DAVID

Sri Satay, good morning.

Satay seemed more amused than concerned about the interruption. It helped that David was nicely dressed and wore a thoughtful, even promising smile. He remained seated. David took a few steps toward him but remained standing behind the chairs in front of the desk.

JEROME

Mr. Skye, isn't it? I think we've met briefly, maybe at a hospital function. Anyway, I can't imagine you are here to waste my time. Please sit down. (Gestures to the chairs) How can I help you? Oh, and by the way, as I think you probably did your research, I am an American. If I use a handle, it is mister.

DAVID

Though you have a doctorate in macroeconomics.

JEROME

(Nods) Please call me Jerome.

DAVID

Thank you, Jerome. Yes, I am David Skye, and I am here not for your gracious offer of help but to provide it to you, and to SMH.

JEROME

I'm impressed and interested. How can you help me?

DAVID

There were three issues at the board meeting the other night during which your position was out-voted even though in each case it was more sound. I would like to suggest how those positions might be presented that they would be recognized for their greater value and affirmed.

JEROME

I'm interested. Impress me.

DAVID

First of all, you only have to change one mind, and you know how his mind works. As with aikido, which I read that you had trained in for a while, you want to blend with him, and he will see that you share his intentions but have a better path to realize them.

That earned David a serious smile.

DAVID

The three issues were vaccinating the staffers, religious exemptions, and the insurance negotiations. Let's start with the religious exemptions. The Supreme Court just validated Maine's denying religious exemptions. But I think UAL handled the matter very well by telling those who claimed exemptions would be furloughed and without pay. It made sense. It worked. When the deadline approached, very few of them held their ground. That should particularly work with the people here since they've seen the alternatives to getting vaccinated, close up and lethally personal. As regards the staffers who are just reluctant or are refusing for other reasons, this isn't about what SMH wants. The federal government is calling for it. More to the point, as with the religious exemptions, your staffers have seen what happens to people who don't get vaccinated. And as has been the case with hospitals across the country that have mandated vaccinations, the great majority decide to get their shots. And it can be made clear that those who don't not only will be let go but they face a seriously problematic future because not only will they have trouble finding any positions in healthcare, but they will be denied unemployment insurance. If that isn't enough, the remaining number will be small, and you won't want them anyway. I would also note that offering regular testing as an alternative to vaccinations would be a mistake. They can be inaccurate, dated, and they're merely an attempt to meet the purpose of limiting contact with the virus.

David paused and looked at Satay who nodded his head.

"As for the insurance situation, disputing who should pick up more of the tab, in a way it's just a public relations issue. You – you meaning the hospital – wouldn't save a ton of money, but it would buy you a great deal of community respect, and respect from the business community for getting more than you have fought for. Because you and the insurance people are really just fighting over money. It's not about healthcare. So why not have the hospital publicly invite the insurance company to agree to split the difference, whatever it is, and put that money to delivering vaccinations to where they are most needed, i.e., the low-income neighborhoods. Yes, the government is paying for the shots, but SMH would set up and man vaccination stations throughout the needy areas.

JEROME

(Silent for more than a minute) Yes, I'm impressed. A question if I might?

DAVID

Of course.

JEROME

You wouldn't be here if you didn't have some muscle behind you. What you told me should be more than enough, and I'd like to see that you don't have to use it. But I wonder what it is.

DAVID

I think what I've said should inform you.

Satay's eyes narrowed slightly in thought. Then they opened with the answer.

JEROME

Very good, yes. One more matter, what do you want from this?

DAVID

(Cocks his head) Just to have it done. If SMH moves in this new direction of very obviously putting health care first on these three points, it will present a new face. Quality management that benefits the community, better delivery of healthcare, and greater attention to the people who work here. They – you – will set a good example for how other hospitals – other businesses should behave.

JEROME

You did do your homework. Thank you for coming to me.

DAVID

Thank you for your time. (Stands, puts his business card on the desk) If you need anything further, please feel free to contact me.

JEROME

(Stands up, comes came around the desk, and offers his hand) We shall meet again, David.

DAVID

I look forward to it, Jerome. (Shakes his hand)

JEROME

And I hope you will bring the charming Ms. Balfour with you.

DAVID

She will be pleased to see you again.

Pharma Accounting

David is driving Lucy to the hospital for her early morning shift.

LUCY

This is my last week, and I am so glad you've gotten most of the information from people there that you think you'll need. Six o'clock is too early to be out of bed. (Smiles to herself; looks at David) Or to be anywhere that is not with you. Thank you for driving me, David.

DAVID

(At a stop light; looks over at her) It's time someone else was missing you and not I.

LUCY

(Laughs) Right on, my darling. And it's good that you're going to see Myrna today.

DAVID

Yes, you told me that Monday morning is when they do their weekly inventory check and the dispensary doors are closed until eight. I won't hold her up but more than fifteen minutes.

Shortly after they arrive at the hospital. Lucy heads for the nurses locker room and David for the dispensary. He knocks on the window as instructed. Myrna Charles raises the window shade, sees David, lowers the shade, and unlocks the door, locking it again when he's inside.

MYRNA

You know this is very much against the rules, but no one of authority ever comes down here at this hour.

DAVID

I'm most appreciative, Myrna. I'll be quick, and as Lucy told you, no one will know that it is you who informed me.

MYRNA

You stay as long as you need, David, ask whatever you want. To tell you the truth, I have moments throughout the day – every day – when I think of quitting, and at least if I was fired, I'd get severance.

DAVID

(Smiles) I can't tell you how many times I've heard that from people here, mostly during the past week or so. What you're going through – everyone here – is terrible and it needs to be straightened out...somehow.

MYRNA

You got that right. So go ahead. Ask me what you want.

DAVID

Great. (Starts micro recorder; holds it facing her) Please tell me in very basic terms how the hospital drugs are managed and controlled, and what are the serious ones.

MYRNA

Okay, right. First of all, every medicine dispensary – hospitals, drug stores, medical practices, whatever – is required to keep careful track of income and outgo of their prescription drugs. Of course. Because there is a considerable number of formulaic prescriptions that can be, and are, used in unprescribed ways. For example, painkillers, including fentanyl, hydrocodone, morphine and oxycodone; barbiturates like Nembutal; benzodiazepines like Valium and Xanax; sedative-hypnotics like Ambien; anti-depressants like Zoloft, Prozac, Lexapro and Paxil. Doctors' offices, which mostly distribute prescriptions, don't handle a lot of drugs so they're allowed little room for error. Drugstores distribute huge amounts of these drugs, and have to be particularly careful that they don't make mistakes because they could be so easily sued in our litigious society. (Looks to David for confirmation)

DAVID

Yes. Good.

MYRNA

Hospitals are different in that they are distributing a considerable amount of different drugs to people that are consuming them on the premises. It's not difficult for the number of pills reported to be going to various patients might be higher than what actually reaches that person. Who would know but the doctor or nurse who delivered the drugs to the patient. What makes the hospital pharma accounting creative is that the diversion of some of the drugs stays in house, so to say. It is for the doctors and nurses who are pushing themselves beyond what most people would see as the limits of endurance. Yes, it would be better if there were more personnel so that the medical folks and all those who back them wouldn't have to work such despairingly long hours, both physically and emotionally straining. Most of the doctors, when they need something for themselves, will ask a colleague to write the script, and they're mostly ready to write for someone when there's no chance – well, little chance – of it being abused. And they'll write for the nurses and some of the staff.

When Lucy needed a prescription drug, she had one of the doctors write it for her. And when you seriously strained your back from moving me into my new apartment...

DAVID

Up those ten flights of stairs...

MYRNA

(Laughs) It was one flight and it was a wide staircase.

DAVID

(Chuckles) Maybe.

MYRNA

So anyway, I had some loose Tylenol with co-deine and I gladly gave them to Lucy for you.

DAVID

I think I only took two, but I was most grateful.

MYRNA

I was grateful to you for getting me away from my idiot roommate and into my place that really feels like my home. I love my private time.

DAVID

Don't we all, Myrna. And we're pleased that you're happy there. You said "loose" about the Tylenol with codeine. What does that mean?

MYRNA

(Smiling) Yeah, that's the big one. When we issue pills and the patient doesn't need to take them all, maybe they're released and they don't take the pills with them, (Winces) or they die, the drugs come back here. Or they're supposed to but may not. But if they do, we can't reissue them and we can't just throw them away. You know that. There is a growing pollution problem being caused by people throwing out drugs or flushing them down the toilet. It's getting into water systems. Some very toxic stuff.

DAVID

(Nods) So you can't just toss them, and I trust you don't sell them on the street....

MYRNA

We go downtown and hand them out to the homeless crowd. No, we keep them out of sight, and distribute them at our discretion. The Tylenol I gave to Lucy for you, she was going to get one of the doctors to write it for you but there was no one available at the time and I insisted she take them.

DAVID

Hah! Now I have something to hang over her head. (Laughs; suddenly curious) But, Myrna, I remember that it had a regular prescription label on it. And a doctor's name.

MYRNA

Doctor Hammett.

DAVID

(Ponders then laughs) Oh my goodness. First name Dashiell? Very cute, Miz Loy. (Shakes his head) Okay, one more question.

MYRNA

Shoot.

DAVID

How have things been different during the pandemic?

MYRNA

(Mood darkens quickly) During crises like the Covid pandemic, and there hasn't been anything so brutal as what we've had to deal with during the past two years, (Sighs) distribution rules had to be bent. Yes, sometimes they were bent too far, but most of the people who come through that door have seen what mistakes can produce. I saw a lot of people who were at the end of their rope, not only for themselves but also for their patients.

DAVID

Were some patients given a faster way out?

MYRNA

(Nods) Yeah. The prescription was legitimate. It was just that too many of the pills were taken at one time. The last time. (Looks hard at David) And yes, sometimes it wasn't the patient who did it.

DAVID

The doctor?

MYRNA

You can't believe the pain they were in...excruciating, and they would never get better. They were gone in hours, maybe a day or two. Why should they suffer?

DAVID

I wouldn't want to. If someone I cared for was suffering with no hope left, I'd help them out if I could. And if it were me, I'd want the same consideration. That's not wrong or bad. It's the right thing for such situations.

MYRNA

(Nods her agreement) I have to tell you, though, so you know the truth, that it wasn't just patients who went early. (Waits for David to understand) There were some overdoses, more than one fatal during the pandemic. It wasn't clear if they were suicides or just mistakes. Either, the relief was real.

DAVID

(Nods) No judgment here, Myrna. I've heard from Lucy, and from what she's heard from others, that people working in the hospitals were taking drugs. Loose drugs?

MYRNA

Probably, but ones they picked up themselves. None from the dispensary...that I personally know of. Pills are found when the bodies are removed. (Deep breath) However they got the pills, finding or sharing, these good people couldn't have gotten through without some help, and their getting that help meant saving the lives of their patients. End of story.

The Icebox

David is sitting under a tent at the end of a row of five freezer trucks, three of them hooked up to a power station to keep the contents at 34 degrees, according to thermometers on the outside at both ends of the trucks. With David are Lescar and Lopez, the two men he drove with in the ambulance.

DAVID

How is it you are doing two jobs?

AMBULANCE DRIVER

The ambulance company only lets us drive ten-hour shifts four days. We're on a different clock here.

AMBULANCE MEDIC

The company got these trucks but they couldn't find the people to, uh, see to the people in 'em. They don't care about us having another job, just so long as they have two guys in the tent, keeping track of the passengers and making sure the freezers are working.

AMBULANCE DRIVER

Also, we have to keep track of the ones that are taken out, you know, families moving them to the mortuaries. Or if there's no known family, down to the city morgue.

DAVID

When did they know that the hospital morgue was not going to be enough?

AMBULANCE MEDIC

They were smart, sort of. April last year, about a month into the pandemic. They were out of space in their morgue in two weeks. They weren't the worst in the area. And they'd already pre-ordered three trucks. Got 'em from a supermarket trucking firm.

AMBULANCE DRIVER

(Chuckles) They got in a big hurry and wanted the trucks sooner, but the supermarket, they had their name on it, they said they had to paint over their name. Cost 'em an extra day.

AMBULANCE MEDIC

Yeah, and when they got here and plugged them in, they found that the power had to be boosted, so it was another half-day. By that time they had the bodies stacked three high in their morgue. They loaded up two trucks full the first night. They only work at night.

AMBULANCE DRIVER

You should have seen them moving two on top of each gurney, racing back and forth. They had to use freezer boxes from the trucking company because they had run out of body bags.

DAVID

I heard they had never seen so many patients dying. Plus so many very sick patients and they were taking up all their beds. Some of the other hospitals were also overloaded and the city had to find ice trucks for them.

AMBULANCE MEDIC

It's bad like they never seen, and we seen the patients comin' and goin'. How's for that? It's really weird. No one's ever seen it like this before.

DAVID

How long do you have the bodies here?

AMBULANCE DRIVER

Yeah, like that's a big problem. The crematories are operating twenty-four/seven. The city told 'em they had to, and they're jammin'. Mortuaries are all backed up. Ya know, it takes time to make the bodies look pretty, and they got to do a lot on the Covid bodies just to have the coffin open. And the cemeteries, they're digging as fast as they can, trying to keep up. Can't get the stones made in time. Dunno when they'll be done.

Into the tent comes a woman in a suit carrying the ubiquitous clipboard atop a stack of files.

MS. ROYAL

(Looks at David) Why Mr. Skye, what are you doing, looking for your nurse lady?

DAVID

Excuse me, you have me at an advantage. I don't think we've met, have we? If we have, please accept my apology.

MS. ROYAL

No need. We were never formally introduced. I'm Meghan Royal. I've seen you dropping off and picking up Nurse Balfour any number of times. I spend a lot of time outside our hospital.

DAVID

Of course, Ms. Royal. Or do you have a title?

MS. ROYAL

Ms. will do just fine. I'm the assistant facilities manager.

DAVID

Well you sure have a heck of a lot on your plate. You asked what I was doing, I know these fellows from their ambulance work. They collected a neighbor of ours a while back when he fell off his ladder when he was clearing his gutters. This was before the pandemic, when the hospital still had the facilities to handle such incidents more easily.

MS. ROYAL

We are gratified to have Mr. Lescar and Mr. Lopez on our team, I can tell you. They are real professionals. They get the job done bringing in the patients, and managing those who don't make it, here in their temporary, next-to-final stops.

DAVID

From what I've seen, the traffic out front and back here, and what my Nurse Lady has been allowed to tell me, HIPAA rules you know, but she's very proud of what you all have been able to accomplish. As difficult as it has gotten. I've also heard from business associates that because

SMH was one of the largest hospitals in the area, and considered highly efficient, it found itself the target for many transfers from other hospitals in the area. That had to have put a significant extra burden on you.

MS. ROYAL

It did, in fact only a matter of days before we had to refuse transfers because we were already overloaded. We even had to set up tents outside in the parking lot. But we had to stop putting up more tents because we didn't have the personnel to treat more patients.

DAVID

Ms. Royal, Santa Marino Hospital is in a rather upscale neighborhood on the border of an expansive metropolitan area. I read that when it was considering locating here, some of the leading residents worked with the founders to make sure that the funding would be enough to hire competent management and staff, and they would be working on up-to-date equipment in a quality facility.

MS. ROYAL

That's right, Mr. Skye. We have built a very good relationship, not only with our neighbors who get first-class medical attention, but throughout the city we have good working relationships with the other hospitals and clinics. This makes for a better healthcare all around. But even those pluses were challenged by the first assault of the coronavirus, and then the subsequent arrival of Delta this past March when hospitals across the United States were reporting full beds and worse.

DAVID

Santa Marino Hospital was also better prepared when Delta hit. I saw that during the relative lull before it struck, the board went on a crash buying program, doubling their precautionary supplies and maintaining those levels. They didn't release the three freezer trucks as the need lessened and disappeared as many hospitals did. Instead, they used them for storage of the extra supplies that needed to be kept cold. That must have added to the length of your work days, Ms. Royal.

MS. ROYAL

(Face shows fatigue) Of course we were all pushed harder, but it needed to be done. Everyone had to put in more hours to get it all done, but we did. Our team worked schedules that many thought were over and above, but we heard little complaining. I'm very proud of our whole SMH team.

DAVID

The board also had the foresight to purchase three funeral homes, at a necessary premium, but they kept all the personnel in place and added more to deal with the influx. That was very smart. Of course, SMH was their primary first client, and the new members of your team made great use of the new facilities. I understand that the board looked at buying a cemetery or starting one, but no one wanted to sell and local permitting requirements were too cumbersome to be practical. So they brought in two more ice trucks and another two thousand body bags from an Israeli military supply firm. That was very forward thinking, Ms. Royal. You must be proud to be working for a board that is ready to write checks for the new facilities and the personnel you need to get the job done.

MS. ROYAL

We couldn't have done what we've done without their foresight and acting, that's for sure.

DAVID

This may not be in your purview, Ms. Royal, but the pandemic has revealed a serious chasm between the states that have fought the virus with masks, social distancing, and mandated vaccinations and those that have blocked those measures. The five states with the lowest vaccination rates – Alabama, Louisiana, Wyoming, Idaho, and Mississippi – are suffering a surge in Delta variant cases.

MS. ROYAL

(Resisting) I think you can appreciate, Mr. Skye, that that is not my area of concern. My focus is right here at Santa Marino Hospital where we are doing all we can to meet the needs of our extended community. And yes, we are very pleased with what we have been able to accomplish, and sorry for not having more space, more people, and more equipment to meet the greater need.

DAVID

Ms. Royal, you know your stuff. Maybe you should be the official spokesperson from Santa Marino. I'm very impressed.

MS. ROYAL

(Slight blush) Well thank you, Mr. Skye. What a nice thing for you to say. But I have my hands full with the facilities. (Smiles) And I'm afraid that I have to get back to my work inside.

DAVID

(Stands) Oh I understand, and again I extend my appreciation and respect for all that you have accomplished and all that you are doing. I wish you the best.

MS. ROYAL

(Pleased, nods) Well thank you again, Mr. Skye. Best to you and your Nurse Balfour.

Ms. Royal walks back toward the hospital.

Lopez and Lescar exchange glances with controlled smiles. David sees it.

DAVID

(Smiles) What did you see?

They exchange the same look.

AMBULANCE DRIVER

You never answered her question.

AMBULANCE MEDIC

She asked what you were doing here and you didn't tell her. Did she forget?

AMBULANCE DRIVER

He didn't let her ask again. Kept her too busy, huh?

DAVID

(Smiles humbly) She didn't need to know. Also, I wanted to make sure you didn't get into any trouble. So gentlemen, I'll get out of here. Thank you.

He hands them both a Franklin.

AMBULANCE DRIVER

Oh, no, Mr. Skye.

AMBULANCE MEDIC

No, we're glad to talk to you. People need to know what's going on here.

DAVID

(Insists) You're doing a great service, especially in the ambulances. It's my way of saying thank you in a personal way.

* * * * *

David and Lucy are sitting on the couch. Music is on in the background. They're each holding a glass of wine. There's a half-full bottle on the table. They have been sharing the highlights of each other's day.

LUCY

That was nice, giving them a hundred dollars each.

DAVID

I also left earlier than I would have if it hadn't been for Ms. Royal. I had a couple more questions, but I was concerned that she might come back and ask them what we talked about or otherwise give them a hard time.

LUCY

She's not a bad egg. But like everyone else, she is badly overworked. Probably eighty hours a week or more.

DAVID

(Whistles) I sense that she was getting a lot done, herding a large number of cats, many with their own problems, light exhaustion or oversized egos.

LUCY

Yes, and judging from the way you stroked her, and the hospital, she would find it personally difficult to try to bring you down. Especially since you wanted to elevate her to an executive job. That was very clever.

DAVID

It's important to recognize and validate the people who are working hard, especially in the lower and middle ranks.

LUCY

You've always been good about that. From the moment we met. When you held me, you the patient and me the nurse.

DAVID

It's funny, Lucy, but not long ago I would have responded with some joke-ish line, but no more. I remember that moment as though it was this afternoon. If you hadn't come to my house at four the next morning, I would have come back to the hospital to get you.

LUCY

Once you were out of the wheelchair, my love.

DAVID

Thank you for saving me from that embarrassing scene. (Leans over; they kiss) And for the most glorious years of my life since. I do love you so, and I'm so glad our being apart will be over at the end of the week.

LUCY

(Leans over; they kiss) Now back to business, if we must. Briefly.

DAVID

Okay, those two new trucks were not needed for

the morgue overflow, but they were used in an unplanned way. For the personnel, I suspect.

LUCY

They were used to recharge batteries. Human batteries. Going through what we were going through left us ragged, as you well know. Anyone who has been through an ongoing crisis that demands every ounce of strength and spirit knows the hungering to have their batteries recharged. They're looking forward like they're in a desert plodding through the sand, knowing there's an oasis up ahead. It's not about miles but hours and then finally minutes 'til they get there. And it saves them. Restores them. It's a promise fulfilled. Just short breaks but they are essential to rebuilding the emotional will to continue the effort. The body might not feel strong enough, but the heart will be there to get the show back on the road. So beds, blankets, and pillows were loaded into the two trucks fixed with low lights for the medical staff to take naps. One truck for the women and one for the men, ostensibly. But they were men and women, and they were emotionally as well as physically exhausted. Battlefield relationships naturally blossomed. They might last minutes or days or even become long-term. There was no way of knowing and under these circumstances, it didn't really matter. One participant said it was like the opium dens of yore – there was no yesterday and no tomorrow, just the very human need to turn off the angst and feel life flowing in their souls.

DAVID

Well said, Lucy. (Pauses) And the top people were aware of what was happening?

LUCY

Of course management had to know. They knew it meant these people, whatever they were doing in those trucks, alone or together, were more likely to be able to function again in the life-saving arena. Some of the people in charge, sharing the twenty-hour shifts, days in a row, are also human.

Lies and More Lies

The sign on the office door reads "Dr. Wendell Mencken, Psychotherapist." Inside the office, the doctor has come out from behind his desk and is sitting across from David in a comfortable chair.

DAVID

Do I have a full fifty minutes, Dell? (Joking)

WENDELL

(Looks at his watch) Forty-nine, David. (Laughs) And how are you, and your wonderful lady? It's been too long since we've had a lengthy dinner together.

DAVID

Wonderful-er every day, my friend. Thank you for asking. And yes, we will be more available soon.

WENDELL

(Hesitates) Hmm. I think I know what that means and I certainly wouldn't press. But may I say I'm very pleased for you both.

DAVID

(Smiling) Thanks.

WENDELL

Now what can I do for you in your remaining time?

DAVID

Dell, I need to get a handle on the misinformation crisis. It seems to be spreading faster than the Delta variant, and I wonder who is spreading it, why, who's buying it, and why. I'd say it doesn't make any sense, but there have to be explanations. I mean, people are not only putting others – including family, friends, co-workers – at risk, but they're also killing themselves.

WENDELL

Some of it is not complicated. It's basically about affiliation. Human beings have an innate need to have relationships with other human beings. They can range from family and friends to parishioners, and sports fans at the favorite bar. Very few people could live without relationships. And they are hard to break. Almost harder to put at risk. That's how important they are.

DAVID

That explains the Trump fandom and the Republican governors going along with him, them. People will buy into false information because they are pre-aligned with a source they won't leave.

WENDELL

That's been particularly strong glue over the past few years. But there's more to it. We have been coming apart as a nation for a long time. I'd put it to the Vietnam war. It was a terrible mistake, and the people who got us into it – our government, the politicians, the military and the media who supported it – never admitted they were wrong, never apologized, and never were punished.

DAVID

I wonder if it doesn't go back further, but the same problem. I look at all the efforts to erase history, taking down Civil War statues, changing the name of Columbus Day, talking about reparations to blacks five generations later. It's chaotic thinking. Or to get into your line of work, it's nuts.

WENDELL

(Takes deep breath; lets it out through his teeth)

Yes it is, and dangerously so. We're not holding people accountable.

DAVID

That's right. All sorts of clamoring for our rights and no one taking responsibility for their errors. I mean, who wants to admit they were wrong. (Thinks) But it has gotten to the point that it isn't that they won't change sides, it seems as though they can't. It's like with the people who won't get vaccinated. They're not making a decision about the vaccine. They're coming up with excuses not to get the shots based on affiliations as you said. Being Republicans, being cops, having those friends at the bar. It's their social associations rather than anything to do with the vaccine. Though they don't admit it.

WENDELL

Yes, you're right, and I haven't heard anyone suggest how the situation can be managed, let alone reversed. (Chuckles) I don't think that's what you came to me to hear.

DAVID

(Pauses) Dell, I want to run something by you that might seem off the wall.

WENDELL

It won't be the first time, though you have rarely

pushed past my limits.

DAVID

Okay. I think what we're dealing with is a global plague of insanity that Mother Nature is using along with climate change and pandemics in her intervention for our failure as stewards of the Earth. And she's aiming to reduce the population by six billion.

WENDELL

(Shakes his head) That doesn't seem off the rails to me at all, David. For a long time, I have been seeing news stories from around the world that have a scent of unreality, and more recently they reek of it. This is your area not mine, but consider Putin, Xi, Duterte, Modi, Netanyahu, Bolsonaro, Orbán, and a dozen other leaders who are successfully undermining the very notion of democracy in democratic countries. (Sighs) The big problem is that it's more than the leaders, it's the populace. There are growing signs of mental instability. At least it's viewed that way by a good many analysts; those with the courage to speak up. One that is very obvious here is the victimhood explosion we talked about the last time we were together. Everyone is claiming to have been wounded or cheated in some way, based on racism, sexism, ageism, and every other ism they can claim to have been hurt by or taken advantage of. And the other, which if you go public with it, will raise a firestorm, is about gender confusion.

DAVID

Meaning not LBGT?

WENDELL

No, though I think a lot of what I'm talking about started there. I mean the people who are having major medical procedures to change their physicality, from what they were born with to the other sex. I think that's over the top, and there's powerful proof that many of the people who are doing this are badly damaged emotionally, to the point that one study said half had considered suicide.

David whistles.

And the anything-goes Democrats aren't raising questions about this movement, they are abetting it. Plus, you surely saw that the State Department is now issuing X Passports so that people don't have to declare their sex. David, you know I am very progressive in my thinking about human rights, but this is lunacy.

DAVID

(Lets out a deep breath) Is there anything to be done about this plague of insanity?

WENDELL

It's a question that keeps me up at night. Because I have two answers, and I'm not sure that I have a preference. Number one is that I'm wrong about the situation and the virus, bad weather, and insanity will all go away. The other is that I'm right, that we need to dramatically reduce the population, that we have to stop polluting the planet, and the crazy people have to take themselves out or we have to.

DAVID

I appreciate the dilemma, my friend, and share the challenge of the choices. Certainly the second one is the noble choice...respect for our dear blue planet Earth and cleaning up the mess that we and our predecessors have made. I mean, if we don't act and quickly, which seems very unlikely considering global politics, we face an end to the Gulf Stream and other basic environmental patterns that will be significantly unsettling, if it's even survivable.

WENDELL

A guy I know quoted a famous professor whose name I forget. Sort of an indictment of what we did and didn't do. He said, "Nature is not nice, not compassionate. She's efficient. Man is the only species that has refused to work with Her."

DAVID

That's worth sharing. Let me know the professor's name if it comes to mind.

WENDELL

I will, certainly, but David, isn't it interesting that probably 99% of the general public would go with door number one and do nothing to make that possible. Leaving us with door number two.

DAVID

That's the yes to rights and no to responsibility mentality. It reminds of something in de Tocqueville's *Democracy in America*. He spoke about a large number of Americans who, rather than raising themselves, would pull down their betters.

WENDELL

Amen in America.

Letters to the Editor

David is sitting in a corner of a hotel bar popular with the Santa Marino media, all but empty at three in the afternoon, but for him and Marty Bevsage, the editorial page editor of the *Santa Marino Star*.

MARTY

My friend, you didn't have to spring for pricey drinks to pick my brain. I always like talking with real journalists.

DAVID

Thank you, Marty. As you know for over how many years we've known each other...

MARTY

Years? Decades.

DAVID

Right, decades. There hasn't been a minute we've

spent together that I didn't find productive, that it didn't make me a better man at the job.

MARTY

Whoa, David. Now I think you're gonna make me buy the expensive hooch.

They laugh.

DAVID

Let's see if you're worth it. First off, I want to congratulate the paper for running such intelligent editorials, at least the ones I've seen, on the pandemic.

MARTY

Any in particular?

DAVID

Yeah, there were a few. I liked the idea that insurance companies shouldn't cover medical costs of Covid patients who refused to get vaccinated. Also, I think hospitals, if they are going to treat anti-vaxxers for Covid, it should be at a premium. I think you even said that the hospital should bar non-vaccinated patients from treatment because they put everyone at risk, including the staffers that might pass along the virus, as well as taking up bed space and treatment three times as much as regular patients. Oh yeah, and my favorite was that the hospital should make a video, maybe a PSA, of the last thirty seconds or a minute of a Covid patient's life, while they try to breathe, their eyes showing fear and the move from life to death, and the last movement of the mouth. It's for the doubters and misinformation cretins to watch. Whatever happened to that idea, anyway?

MARTY

Whaddya think? They didn't have the guts to produce it. I've seen that stuff. A nurse shot the deaths of several of her patients. Lousy video but oh my god, it told the story, undeniably gory. (Shakes his head) Don't remind me. Tell me what's up? Your email said you were wondering what kind of hee-haw we're getting in the letters about Covid.

DAVID

Yes, especially the excuses for not getting vaccinated and also any weird stuff, like plugs for ivermectin.

MARTY

What are you doing with it, if I might ask?

DAVID

You can always ask, Marty, and I will always tell you. Especially now, because you know how important Lucy is to me.

MARTY

Important? That girl is everything to you. I don't know anyone who knows you two who isn't respecting of your relationship to seriously jealous.

DAVID

(Smiles his thanks) Yes, well she has finally decided she's had enough, and she's given notice.

MARTY

Smart. My blessings upon her, and you both.

DAVID

Thanks. In talking about it, the idea came up that she might help me get information about what Covid has done to the hospital – the people who work there, the patients, dealing with the death, et cetera.

MARTY

(Nods) That could be big.

DAVID

From what I've gotten already, it is. Some of it, as you would imagine, is very poignant.

MARTY

And what you asked me for will add some bright

colors to the dreary facts.

DAVID

(Chuckles) I hadn't thought of it in quite those terms but yes.

MARTY

(Pulls out his phone; finds a file) We get a ton of stuff. It's been flooding us since about a week into the pandemic. So much that I had to pull in an assistant to screen them first. Not taking out the craziest. It is important that the public get a smell of just how nutty some of the people out there are.

DAVID

And that's just among the people who write to you. I'm not sure if that's good or scary.

MARTY

(Shakes his head) It's scary either way. We've added security to our building and fine-tuned our cyber ops.

DAVID

I was talking with Dell Mencken the other day. He is deeply concerned about what's happening, not just over Covid but the social collapse here and around the world.

MARTY

(Serious) We are talking about that amongst ourselves almost every day, seeing the headlines we see; some from the wire services that we don't print. We're regularly revisiting our approach – what we are going to report and our tone.

DAVID

Blessings upon you, my friend. Do stay safe. It's insane that we have reason to have this conversation.

MARTY

Yeah, so let me read to you some of the better stuff we're getting. Then I'll send you a file that you can pick from.

DAVID

Good. And I won't refer to the *Star*. You don't need any further hassle.

MARTY

Appreciate. Okay. Here are some of the excuses we're heard. "You become a zombie....Only dogs get vaccinated.... I don't have the virus so I don't need it. ...The vaccine makes you magnetic.... I don't know all the ingredients....I use a hand sanitizer and it's the same thing....God will protect me....It'll make men/women sterile....An old truck driver told me not to....The vaccines are too new." Oh, and one of favorites: "A microchip, with the backing of Bill Gates, is being implanted with the vaccine."

DAVID

I heard that one yesterday from a friend I hired for my newsroom fifteen years ago. She tied it to 5G somehow. Also, she said that being a libertarian, she didn't feel the government had the right to tell her what to do.

MARTY

(Shaking his head) Okay, now for some of really crazy stuff. You mention ivermectin. We have heard from a number of people that the livestock de-wormer works better than the vaccines. These are all people in the good old USA.

Televangelist Elvin Coppleman told his followers to touch their televisions when he was on, and they would be vaccinated by proxy. He also did exorcisms to get rid of Covid-19 in whoever was watching. Did at least three of 'em, saying he was summoning "the wind of God."

Number two was "Joyous Life" which is some kind of secretive, pay-to-play religious group, that sells "spiritual vaccines" to prevent and cure Covid-19. They also sell virus-related blessings starting at $100 and go to over $400. I haven't a clue what the differences are.

Here's one you'll like. Remember the TV preacher Jim Bakker? Of course you do. Well the state of Missouri is suing him for selling a product called Silver Sol Liquid that he claimed could diagnose and cure Covid-19.

And then there's this Genesis II Church of Health and Healing in Florida. A federal court ordered them "to stop promoting their own concoction, master mineral solution, or MMS, as a cure for Covid-19." Apparently MMS contains chlorine dioxide, and they say drinking the stuff according to their directions is like "drinking bleach."

DAVID

God help us.

MARTY

Probably not. And from abroad, various third world leaders in particular – and you wouldn't recognize their names – have promoted vodka, cognac, and other alcohol drinks to "play a major role in killing the coronavirus."

Also, there's an Indian swami who says that drinking cow urine and applying cow dung on the patient's body will cure Covid-19. But he said it that only works with Indian cows.

DAVID

Oh good. I was finding that tempting.

MARTY

Staying six feet apart wouldn't be enough, I don't think.

They laugh.

MARTY

Oh and if it's more convenient, maybe you want to drink camel urine which has been advocated in the Middle East.

DAVID

Good grief. It's just appalling.

MARTY

It's worse than that. You keep seeing the stories about Facebook and Twitter being the source of so much misinformation, and they frickin' knew better.

DAVID

There was a piece I saw yesterday, you probably saw it, about the "Disinformation Dozen" who were found responsible for 65% of the disinformation on Twitter and Facebook over 45 days last winter. And on Facebook alone those twelve were found responsible for 73% of the anti-vaccine content.

MARTY

David, they've got blood on their hands.

Payoff

David and Lucy are having dinner with Jerome Satay in a private dining room of a swank restaurant. Sitting chatting while waiting for the wine and appetizers.

JEROME

I'm so pleased that you could make it on such short notice, David and especially, if I might say so, Lucy. I've learned that you will be leaving us in the very near future.

David ostentatiously looks at his watch. They laugh.

LUCY

My last shift is tomorrow, starting at eight. With any luck, I'll be off at four.

JEROME

Is there going to be a going-away party?

LUCY

I said no, not now. Too many of my colleagues –

my friends – were going to be working, if not one shift then another. I said I would plan a party for all of us after this insane pandemic is over. As soon as we can live normal lives, except for the memories.

JEROME

That sounds more reasonable.

Two bottles of wine, the red already decanted, are brought to the table along with six wine glasses. The sommelier looks to Jerome who looks him a yes and pours the wines into the glasses.

JEROME

Thank you. May I offer a simple toast? (Sees nods; holds up glass) To a new start.

Lucy and David look at each other with smiles. They all drink.

DAVID

That sounds very encouraging, Jerome.

JEROME

I am encouraged. I spoke with Abel this morning. That's why this invitation was so late. He listened well to what I relayed from you (Raises glass to David) on the three points you spoke about to me. He was clearly impressed. He began to tell me how pleased he was to have me on the board.

That the ideas were top drawer – Abel is Ivy League – and he wanted me to work closer with him for the benefit of the hospital.

DAVID

How wonderful.

LUCY

Indeed. (To David) Truly wonderful.

DAVID

I gather he thinks there wouldn't be any difficulty with the board to move forward on them.

JEROME

(Pauses) I won't say that Abel *is* the board but with the enthusiasm he showed for all three new directions, each one at a time, the sun will shine.

DAVID

Thank you so much for this, Jerome.

JEROME

(Holds up his hand to David; smiling) There's more.

Lucy and David look with curious interest but no worry.

He asked how I had arranged my mind to come up with these approaches as they seemed similar in tone.

LUCY

Oh really. Excuse me, I wouldn't have expected that from him. Good, good for him.

JEROME

Yes. (Looking at David; holding back a smile) Not the man you saw on the video, I think.

DAVID

I am as delighted with him, with you, Jerome, and of course (turning toward Lucy) with this marvelous woman who was the impetus behind it all.

Lucy blushes. Leans toward him and they share a quick kiss.

LUCY

Thanks to all of you.

The appetizers arrive and the service captain serves the six different tastes onto their plates. They wait until he is finished to resume the conversation.

JEROME

Where was I? (Pretending) Oh yes. I was saying that Abel wanted to know how I had sourced these great ideas. And I told him that I sat quietly at my desk... (Looks at David) as you were telling me what I had told him.

David and Lucy are smiling.

Needless to say he was very impressed.

David nods his appreciation.

Which brings me to another matter that I wanted to raise with you. Abel asked me to offer you a seat on the board.

DAVID

(Surprised but not interested) That's very nice, Jerome, and Abel. (Looks at Lucy who knows David's answer). Very gracious. (Sighs) But Jerome, that's not my venue. I'm a journalist. I feel any formal affiliation would be inappropriate. Thank you, but I hope you and the chair will appreciate my reason for turning you down.

JEROME

(Looks at David for a short while) I can't say I'm surprised, David. I understand your position and appreciate your professionalism.

David nods. Looks at Lucy who smiles back.

I have to tell you that you were my second choice, David.

His tone mitigates any concern for forthcoming explanation.

I must tell you that I expected this would be your

position and I am not disappointed at your decision. I also think we will always have access to
your wisdom. Especially because I think you'll
support our first choice for the seat. (Looks at
Lucy) You, Lucy.

LUCY

(Surprised) What?.. I...Me?

DAVID

(Had seen it coming) Brilliant. First of all, her
experience. Second because she's a much better
human being than I am; far more patient.

LUCY

But David, that's not my thing.

DAVID

Darling, after four o'clock tomorrow afternoon
you won't have a thing.

All laugh.

LUCY

Oh my goodness. Of course I'm flattered. Startled
and flattered. But I'm not sure. (Looks at David;
he raises his eyebrows over his smile) (To Jerome)
Do I have any time to think about it?

JEROME

Of course. (Looks at his watch)

David and Jerome laugh; she joins them.

LUCY

We can eat first?

More laughter.

LUCY

Thank you.

*   *   *   *   *

A montage of the dinner that is served and consumed with lots of conversation, interest, smiles, friendship. After-dinner drinks have been poured and drunk.

JEROME

So, you've eaten.

LUCY

Yes, the whole evening, Jerome, has been delicious.

JEROME

(Chuckles) But I can't imagine that you were spending a lot of time thinking about my invitation for you to join the board of directors.

LUCY

(Smiles) You are such a gracious host, and you were right. I didn't spend a lot of time considering your most honoring offer. But I must decline.

I need a clean break from where I've been and what I've been doing.

Jerome is somewhat disappointed but not greatly surprised. David is not surprised and not at all disappointed.

But I have an alternative offer which might meet your purpose as well, both my thoughts on what the board might be considering, and David's too. I think he would agree to us getting together privately and unofficially to talk about the issues that warranted outside attention.

David shows his pride and affection to Lucy.

JEROME

My goodness, Lucy, that's a fine alternative. Good for you. And David, you seem to like it.

David and Lucy smile and nod to each other.

In fact, I like it so much, I'm inclined to follow that path and resign my seat from the board. Then we could have dinner once a month and I could feed the input from the three of us to Abel. (Chuckles) Between us, those meetings are lengthy and often very boring. It's no one's fault really, but it's quite inefficient. Good. I'll speak with Abel. He may join us.

Laughter.

___The Chapel of Tears___

David is sitting in his car in a parking space near the nurses exit door. He looks at the dashboard clock. It's just four o'clock. He smiles, looks up, and sees Lucy standing in the doorway. She waves and gestures for him to come to her. He gets out of the car and walks to the door. She throws her arms around him.

LUCY

Oh, darling you can't imagine how happy I am to see you.

DAVID

(Concerned) Is everything all right, Lucy?

LUCY

Everything is fine. Wonderful. I want you to come with me for a few minutes, and then we can go home.

DAVID

Sure, sweetheart.

He enters. She takes his arm and leads him down the

hall.

Where are we going?

LUCY

(Squeezes him) You haven't been here before, David.

He doesn't have to know but then his eyes see a sign above a door to which she is directing him that reads, Chapel.

Just a few minutes, please, David.

DAVID

(Squeezes) Of course, my love.

He opens the door for her and follows her in. It isn't a large room. The front area has no religious symbols but is dressed in fresh flowers. There are sets of pews on either side of an aisle; places for maybe forty people. There is some soothing instrumental music playing quietly; again no religious themes.

There are only three people there, all in hospital attire, spread widely around. Lucy gently directs them into the back row. They sit, holding hands, looking forward at nothing in the direction of the flowers.

After five minutes, David looks at Lucy to see tears on her face. His face shows an inclination to offer her warmth and caring but he doesn't want to intrude.

A few minutes later, Lucy sniffs. She takes a handkerchief from her bag and wipes away the tears and touches her nose. She looks up at David, smiling, and nods. They both stand up and quietly leave the chapel. Wordlessly, her arm through his, they walk down the hallway to the exit. David opens the door for her and they walk over to the car.

DAVID

Is there anything you need from me, Lucy? Anything I can do for you?

She shakes her head. Smiles at him.

LUCY

Maybe unlock the car?

David opens the car door for her and gestures as if he might help her in. She puts her arms around him and holds him for a long moment before she lets him go.

LUCY

Thank you, David. I love you.

She releases him and gets into the car. He closes her door, circles around and gets in the other side. He looks at her to assure himself that she needs nothing more here. Then he starts the car and drives off.

LUCY

I don't know if you were surprised that I wanted to go to the chapel. I mean, you know that I'm not a religious person.

DAVID

Yes, but you are one of the most spiritual people I've ever known. And I wasn't surprised. I was just glad to be with you there.

LUCY

(Smiles warmly) Appropriately, my dearest love. It was the first time I think I've been there in all my years at the hospital. I think you could see how little draw there is there. Not faulting the hospital, but it's to serve people of all different affiliations.

DAVID

I think we bring our own beliefs to such a place.

LUCY

That's right. (Quiet) Do you know what I was doing there, David?

David thinks, then shakes his head.

I wanted... (Chokes; clears her throat) I felt a need... Because I wanted to say goodbye. To all of the people I took care of. Those who walked out, and those who didn't.

Tears roll down her cheek. She sobs. David pulls a handkerchief from his pocket and hands it to her. She takes it with a nod of thank-you, uses it on her face, and blows her nose. David gently rubs her shoulder.

No more words are spoken the last two minutes of the ride home. When they arrive, Lucy waits until David opens her door, and they walk hand in hand toward their front door. She stops about ten feet away and turns to David.

LUCY

We're home, David. Finally, and forever together.

About the Author

Tony Seton is a journalist, writer, and publisher. An Emmy award-winning broadcast journalist for ABC Television News, he covered Watergate, six elections, and five space shots. And he produced Dan Cordtz's business/economics coverage and Barbara Walters' news interviews.

Later, Tony wrote and produced two award-winning public television documentaries.

Through Seton Publishing, Tony has written, designed, and published more than 50 of his own books and screenplays, and has edited and published 30-some books for clients.

As a political consultant, his clients have included Nancy Pelosi, Tom Campbell, John Vasconcellos, the American Nurses Association, and various local candidates.

He has taught journalism and writing, provided media training, and produced websites.

Tony is also a private pilot and a photographer.

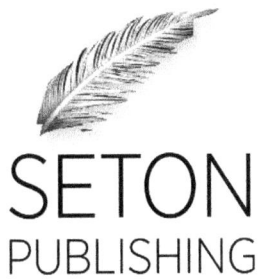

SETON
PUBLISHING